THE JOURNEY

The Journey to Recovery after a Stroke

by

Sharmilah Begum Mehmood

THE JOURNEY

Table of Contents

Message From The Author

Welcome to the Journey. This is a short story about my 3 years of living with a stroke.

I hope my book will motivate you to take care of your health so that you can enjoy a pain-free lifestyle.

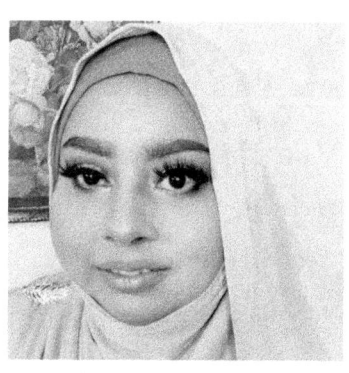

There are ordinary things in life that we take for granted until these are taken away from us.

These includes the act of breathing, the gift of sight, the pleasures of walking, enjoying good food with a fine taste bud, and the independence of travelling anywhere unaided.

At a time when I don't seem to have anything to offer to anyone, I see the true colors of people. To those who are kind to me, I appreciate your kindness and friendship.

You can reach me at sharmilah.begum2019@gmail.com

Keep in touch!

The Day that Changed My Life.

May 18, 2017, 12 midnight. The clock struck and the stroke hit me suddenly. And my life changed forever.

Moments before it happened. I was feeling thirsty, so I went to the kitchen to get myself a glass of water. As I was sitting at the dining table, I saw a figure in white passing by the curtains and going up the stairs.

I felt an evil presence in the air, couldn't make it out but something horrendous was glaring at me. I was feeling giddy and confused so I made my way to bed.

My right arm was in pain. My hands felt like it had a life of it's own, extraordinarily strong and looked kind of evil. My right hand tried to strangle me. My left hand was pulling my right hand back. In my confused state of mind, I said a prayer. Slowly I felt my left hand releasing it's grip of my right arm. Then my right arm and both my legs became numb...paralyzed! It was so bizarre!

Stroke...but I didn't have a clue!!!

As I needed to ease myself, I tried to get up to go to the toilet but I fell to the floor instead. Try as much as I could, I just didn't have the strength to bring myself to stand and walk, so I crawled to the toilet in my room and managed to lift myself up to the toilet bowl, eased myself, washed up and crawled back to my bed.

I asked God for the strength to lift myself on to the bed. After the struggle of lifting myself on to the bed which seemed like an eternity, I fell asleep almost immediately. A few hours later I woke up and realized that I was paralyzed.

I dialed 995 and in my slurry speech, managed to give them the address. The person who took my call knew immediately that I was having a stroke…the signs were there. "Ma'am, you're having a stroke, you're slurring, don't worry Ma'am just stay calm, I've already dispatched an ambulance for you". Kudos to that person!

The ambulance took me to Tan Tock Seng Hospital. I was under observation for 6 hours before being admitted to the neurology ward.

Later that evening, while laying in bed with my boyfriend beside me, I had another stroke, only this time it was a massive one! I passed out. Within minutes, I was wheeled out for a MRI scan. The doctors found a clot, had to remove it immediately!

Lucky for me, I was warded and under observation as it's a well known fact that for stroke cases, treatment should be within three hours!

One of the neurologists met with my boyfriend and told him that "I had to be operated on immediately"…and also said "it is a massive one, she might end up as a vegetable even after the operation, whatever it is…we need to do the op now!"

After the MRI scan while I was being wheeled to the operating theatre to remove the clot in my brain, I had an out-of-body experience. I saw myself laying on the bed, my boyfriend was there beside me crying like a baby. Then, I saw myself walking in a barren hot deserted place. I asked myself, "Am I going to hell…but why? I did lots of good deeds, charity work. I fed the poor. I fed stray cats. I provided shelter for those who were homeless. Why am I going to hell…why not heaven?

About 12 hours later after the operation, I woke up in ICU and saw my brother and my sister-in-law by my bedside.

A short while later, a doctor came in and said, "Sharmilah, your body is in a mess. If you don't take action after this, I don't think you can live for long."

This is not something I wanted to hear after what I've just gone through.

My Body was Failing

Half paralyzed now, I was warded for two weeks. The doctor said that if I am not healed within the next 6 months, my condition will be permanent.

I underwent physiotherapy. I fought my fears with prayers. I called upon God as I took each step.

My organs were failing me. The pain was so excruciating that I could not bring myself to sleep.

To rub salt to the wounds, I had a clot in my heart. I needed to get rid of it or I could have a heart attack …anytime. My heart was a ticking time bomb!

My eyes were bleeding internally because of the blood thinner I took after the stroke.

My kidneys were failing me too.

My feet were in constant pain and the doctors recommended an intensive and painful reconstructive surgery of my right foot. The probability of recovery is 80%...but in the worst case scenario if there was an infection, they may have to amputate my leg.

I went for eye operations for both my eyes.

Gradually, I recovered. My boyfriend was praying for me and with me. God heard his prayers and saw his tears. His undying passion, compassion and dedication made me want to fight for another chance to live. His love and support helped me to recover.

But sometimes when the pain gets too much and my challenges are beyond my control, I whisper to myself, "Should have just died rather than to survive this stroke and live like a handicap."

I felt like the living dead. I want to die but I can't die. I want to live but I can't live.

My Eyes

When the doctor told me, I might go blind due to Diabetic Retinopathy, my whole world collapsed. I cried uncontrollably.

What is life without sight? I lost my motivation to do business, to pursue my dreams...and even to live! Everything that I had built in my life was a waste of time. I could not think anymore. I just wanted to vanish from the face of the earth.

Each time during the laser treatment, it felt like thousands of pins were pricking my eyeballs leaving behind a faint burning smell. I was awake the whole time during each treatment. I could see what the eye surgeon was doing.

The only comforting part was the eye surgeon was a good-looking hunk that made me forget about the pain and fear I was going through.

After each treatment, my sights were blurred, I had to put on dark glasses to protect my eyes from the glares of the sun. Back then I was still single, no boyfriend to pick me up or send me home... no choice but to find my way back home...alone.

I went for many more rounds of the laser treatments, for a year at least, until the doctors told me that they cannot do the treatments anymore!

The Effects of Self-Medication

The pharmacist gave me a big plastic bag full of medicine. I have never liked taking medication. No one does.

The reason why my health deteriorated was, because in the beginning stages when I was diagnosed with diabetes and high blood pressure, I went against the doctors advice and ditched all my medication for supplements.

I was wrongly advised by so-called supplements experts with no medical background. They convinced me that the supplements can reverse my condition. I thought I was smart and well read. I foolishly believed in them.

It turned out that the supplements actually did more harm than good to my body. Each time I took supplements I would have uncontrollable diarrhea.

One day my body started reacting, in fact it over reacted. I had diarrhea non stop, 89 times! I called for an ambulance. I was extremely worried because my bowels were 'exploding' non-stop!

The paramedics handled the situation well. The nurses at the hospital kept changing diapers after diapers. I was afraid to eat or drink for fear of my bowels 'exploding' again!

I stayed in the hospital for 2 weeks.

I felt so vulnerable and embarrassed because the nurses had to clean me each time…like a baby! I wished I could have just disappeared. I had to be on adult diapers all the time. It felt so degrading.

But the nurses were like angels. They cleaned me up. They said that it was normal to be sick. They comforted me.

I wrote to the CEO of the hospital to thank the nurses for their kindness and professionalism so that they would receive the due recognition. I am especially thankful for two Filipina nurses who were both like Florence Nightingale.

The Effects of Warfarin

After the stroke, the doctors gave me Warfarin, which is a blood thinner. But every time I took Warfarin, I felt weak, disoriented, and breathless.

My speech was slurred and I felt uneasy speaking to anyone because people would not understand what I was trying to say.

I drooled a lot while eating and my mucus was uncontrollable.

I get emotional easily. I felt a rage in me. If I did not manage my emotions, I would sink into depression. I felt like I could slide into a psychotic state and hurt myself.

My doctor said that I have to be on Warfarin for life. If I stopped taking it, I might have internal injuries.

But without the doctor's permission I decided not to take the Warfarin because I did not like the side effects of feeling weak, disoriented and breathless!

However, upon stopping the medication, one thing led to another...my legs started swelling...and a clot was found in my heart!

I was admitted to the hospital yet again. Through a scan, they detected the clot. My heart could stop anytime because of that tiny little clot!

I told the doctor to stop the Warfarin. He was furious! He said "Are you aware that the clot appeared only because you stopped taking the Warfarin?"

I told him that I was always in a psychotic mood after taking Warfarin.

He replied "You don't have a choice!". Imagine my frustration.

Warfarin is a blood thinner; it helps blood flow smoothly through the veins and arteries. It also keeps clots from forming or getting bigger.

Okay, now that I'm back on Warfarin everything was going to be under control...or so I thought. No, my eyeballs started to bleed internally!!!

I had to make a choice. Stop Warfarin, ignore the clot and save my eyes or continue with Warfarin, save my heart and lose my eyes?

How do you make such a choice? Had to continue with Warfarin!

Not long after, I couldn't see, everything was blurred. I went for countless eye checks and two eye surgeries. After surgery my left eye regained perfect vision but my right eye was in an advanced stage of Glaucoma for which there was no known cure...yet.

Through prayers and medicine, a miracle happened, the clot in my heart disappeared and the doctor said my heart is normal again.

But...I lost vision in my right eye.
Big is Gorgeous

I blame my poor health on my eating habits. I am an emotional eater.

I blame it on my ignorance. I don't remember learning anything about healthy eating in school.

Back then did they really teach us or could it be that maybe I was not paying attention?

All I remember is, we were taught how to make rock buns. Buns that were really hard as rock, hence the name. It was more like a weapon, not a bun! It was rumored that walls might crack and faces might get disfigured if thrown at them!

Once, I went out with a lady for dinner. A gentleman who was observing us came over to our table and said that I was beautiful, radiant and full of confidence for a plus-size lady. I replied that it was because I was happy with myself, happy with who I am.

After he left, the lady that was with me gave me a glare and said in a furious tone "no woman can be happy in that obese body of yours! Stop lying to yourself! You're just giving excuses not to exercise and lacked discipline in your food intake. Soon you'll have boils popping up due to your sugar issue!"

She was right, I did have boils popping out in no time. I felt confused, could she be right? Maybe I was putting up a false facade to cover up my suffering. Not long after that, I had two carbuncles aka boils, one at the front and the other at the back of my head. To get rid of them, I had to go for surgery…twice!

Her words angered me, I felt she was being judgemental, especially towards plus size women! So, I decided to start a movement for plus size women and I called it B.I.G – 'Big Is Gorgeous'

'Big Is Gorgeous' is a movement to empower plus size women through fashion, catwalk, nutrition and dancing.

Today when I look back, I think it was a mistake, BIG was a mistake. Yes, being big is gorgeous only if you eat healthy and live healthy.

Medically it has been proven that if you are obese, you are bound to suffer depression. People tend to hide the depression behind a smile, so it goes undetected

Today when I see plus size activists campaigning for such body positive movement, I wish I could tell them that they are sending all the wrong messages.

There is nothing positive about it!

If I could do it all again, I will, I will do it all differently!

Money Worries

You can imagine how my medical bills were piling up. I had no insurance. There was little in my Medisave account. My savings were gone. How am I going to pull through?

My only hope is God and by faith. I surrendered completely to Him. He is my Healer, my Provider, and my Protector.

God heard my prayers and sent the government as one of my Guardian angels. The government has put in place a great system for people in the same predicament like what I was going through. I was assured that I will get the necessary treatment, specialist and my bills will be covered by MediFund.

MediFund is a Government safety net that provides partial or full financial assistance to needy Singaporeans, so that they can have access to clinically appropriate care regardless of ability to pay.

I am grateful the government provides for me through the Medifund even though I did not have insurance coverage.

I was diagnosed with Diabetes Type 2 when I was 20 years old and when I turned 21, I tried to buy insurance for myself but no insurance company wanted me even when I was willing to pay a higher premium. I was living in fear constantly. I was worried about my high medical costs as my Medisave was insufficient. I felt my life was like walking on thin ice.

My second worry was the loss of income as I was not able to work anymore.

How am I going to live with no income? The government gives me $500 every month along with free medical treatment.

For transport, the heavily subsidized ambulance ferry service provided by the Red Cross, ferries me to the hospital and back every fortnightly for check ups.

Another great thing the government has done for me is, they allowed me to withdraw my money from my CPF account. But I am not doing so because that money would come in handy in the future when I buy a house.

The government also provides either a motorized or normal wheelchair for free if I ever needed one.

I went to the handicapped center once. They tried assisting me in finding jobs to suit my disability. My only concern was not being able to take public transport like buses and MRT on my own. The center said that they would arrange for my taxi fares, provided by the government. But with me being blind in one eye and my legs being swollen all the time, I can't travel on my own…I need help to move around.

After being discharged from the hospital, my bills came up to $30k but I went home with peace of mind because the government had fully paid for my bills..

The Greed for Money

When I was hospitalized, I was disgusted with the families of some of the patients.

I saw a groups of different generations spending time with sickly elderly patients.

I was thinking they must love the patient so much.

But sadly, they were actually discussing the will, CPF monies, property, insurance and inheritance.

How insensitive of them to talk about it in front of the patient. Instead of caring for the patient, they were more concerned on their share and distribution of the so-called wealth!

In a way, I think it is good of our government to control our parent's CPF monies otherwise the children would have spent it all.

During my hospital stay I have met some elderly patients who didn't have any visitors. I sat with them and it really saddened me to listen to their stories.

Some of them had no savings or property because they have given all their assets and money to their children …after which the children simply forgot about them.

The Empress Dowager

As I laid on the hospital bed recuperating. I was very worried. Being single, I enjoyed being independent. But now I have to depend on others to take care of my every needs.

I thought I should live in a nursing home so that I do not have to burden other people.

My best friend came and she said she will hire a maid for me and I can stay with her.

My second sister asked me to let her do her duty as a sister. In the past, I have helped her and her children. She promised she will do her best to care for me.

At that moment, I felt that my good deeds have translated into good karma.

After 2 weeks of stay in the hospital, I was discharged.

I stayed with my sister and her children. I wondered if they would get frustrated taking care of me.

In the first week, I was a mess. I was still paralyzed. I could not control my bowels. I defecated around the house. My nieces and nephews calmed me down. They helped me to the toilet. They washed me up and showered me

God had sent angels in the form of my nieces and nephews. They dressed me up and made me comfortable. They lovingly took care of me.

I had to wear adult diapers. Diapers were expensive. A good adult diaper could cost up to $5 apiece. Sometimes I needed two pieces a day.

A few months later my eldest sister decided to be my caregiver. I went over to her place to stay with her.

Back then, my mother who is suffering from dementia, was living in Malaysia. My sister went over to Malaysia and brought her back to Singapore so she could look after both my mother and me.

When I saw my mother's condition, I was heart-broken. I cried often. I felt sorry for my eldest sister who had to take care of both my mother and me...two needy adults.

My mother needs to urinate every half hour.

Even though with swollen feet and a weak arm, I brought her to the toilet. I was afraid that I would fall as I could not balance my weak legs but I still accompanied her.

When I slept with her, I was worried that she might wander off or fall in the middle of the night. I kept waking up to check on her every now and then. It was so stressful for me that I fell sick often.

I was admitted to the hospital for 2 weeks. The doctor said that I might suffer a stroke again. My kidney was failing.

My future looked bleak and hopeless.

After a few months of living with my eldest sister, my brother asked me to come and live with him as he has a helper who can help look after me too. He cried. His heart was so broken to see me in this pathetic condition. He asked me not to refuse him as I have helped him a lot in the past and now it was time to reciprocate my kindness.

Dementia is not easy to deal or live with so my sister thought it would be better for my mother to be placed in a nursing home where proper professional care could be given to her. It was a painful decision but it had to be done.

With time, I began to look at life positively.

At first, I hated it when I lost my independence to shower and dress myself up. Then it hit me, I was like living the life of an Empress Dowager.

When the Empress Dowager needed a shower, the courtesans would prepare her bath. They would shower her and dress her up.

Meals have to be prepared and served to her at all times. When she walks, someone has to hold her hands or be around her. She is escorted at all times.

When I needed something, I just asked for it. I get priorities in public places. I can cut the queue. Sometimes strangers will offer me help.

I thought to myself. I am not handicapped. I am living an Empress

Dowager's lifestyle. Whatever the universe has thrown at me, I might as well be happy about it.

Anxiety Attack

Warfarin gave me lots of anxiety. When I traveled alone in a taxi for my regular hospital check-ups, I get anxiety attacks. I would cry and the driver would panic. I told them to just send me to the hospital. Sometimes while travelling I would vomit.

My hospital visits were once every 2 weeks to see the either the stroke doctor, heart and kidney doctor, orthopedic, or the diabetes doctor.

At that point, I have not received help yet from the Red Cross. So I went alone for my check-ups with my walking stick.

My eyes were not blind yet. Still manageable.

I did not ask for help from my family members as I didn't want to trouble them to take leave from their work just to accompany me.

The taxi drivers were helpful when they drove me to the hospital. They gently helped me in and out of their taxis. The drivers would ask the porters to assist me with a wheelchair and informed them I was alone.

The porters would bring me to the registration counter, then hand me over to the nurse or the doctor. After my check-ups, the porters would help me to settle my payment and help me to collect my medications. They would then help push my wheelchair to the taxi stand. When I reached my block, I would call either one of my family members to pick me up. If I was strong enough to walk, I would go up on my own but very rarely as I was afraid I would fall.

My anxiety attacks affected my sleep. I was scared to sleep at night. I was afraid that the stroke would happen again. I was constantly living in fear. I could not be left alone at home.

My Encounter with a Chinese 'Uncle'

One early morning, I decided to go to the park where a few old aunties were exercising.

Even though I was younger than all the old aunties, I didn't have the strength or stamina to exercise, I felt sad and ashamed that the aunties had more stamina than me.

I sat down and look around. I looked up to the sky and whispered to myself, *"Dear God, will I ever get healing from you?"*

Then out of nowhere, a Chinese Uncle came and sat next to me. He was singing an Indonesian dangdut song. The song released the once bubbly and happy-go-lucky Sharmilah...so I sang along with him.

My spirit was lifted. I felt so hearty and I stood up to make my way home.

The uncle asked me what happened to me. Why was I walking with a walker at such a young age? I told him what happened and he said, "I can try to heal you if you would let me..."

He introduced himself as Mr.Ng, David Ng...a retired Chinese physician.

"I cannot afford to pay you", I replied.

He said. "I don't want your money. Just a cup of coffee at the Kopitiam across the road is enough."

I felt God heard me.

There and then, he applied pressure on some points of my paralyzed arm and I could actually feel the blood flowing again. It was painful when he pressed my arm. I screamed in silence.

For the next 6 days, he came over every day to massage my arms. He also brewed some natural concoction for me to consume daily.

After the stroke, I had difficulty shampooing, combing my hair or dressing up by myself. I was always feeling cold, even on a hot day. I had to always cover myself with a blanket.

But after his treatment, my hands and arms were able to function better and I could dress myself up and shampoo my hair. My body felt warm again. No more feeling cold all day and night. The swelling on my leg subsided.

What it Feels like to be a Diabetic

Let me bring you on a journey of what it feels like to live in a diabetic body.

You have a strong craving for sugar. You will need the fix otherwise you'll feel nauseated.

You are constantly thirsty, lethargic, and extremely sleepy.

You feel sluggish and people will think you are lazy. They don't understand.

Depression will hit you and you'll feel very emotional most of the time. Your feelings are easily bruised.

If you don't eat on time, you will have low sugar which makes you giddy or you'll feel like you're about to faint. Your tummy and hands will start to tremble.

Since you are always thirsty, you will drink a lot and no amount of water will quench your thirst. You will urinate a lot and often.

But if you took your medication, all these will be under control.

One day while sitting in the office, I realized my right leg was swollen.

I went to see the doctor. He said that it was due to prolonged uncontrolled diabetes, my nerves were damaged. It was so painful to walk with swollen feet. My shoes were very tight when my feet swelled.

Every night I cried myself to sleep. My legs felt heavy. Walking was physically torturing but despite all that, I was still teaching belly dancing…5 hours a day. I was suffering in silence.

High Blood Pressure

During my hospitalization, the doctor prescribed Glipizide, a diabetes medication. I noticed a tremendous improvement in my blood sugar. My reading was usually in the 20's but Glipizide brought it down to a low of 6.

When you have high blood pressure, you're always feeling tired, in a bad mood and feeling disoriented. You'll have constant headaches and you're always sleepy. Your shoulders will feel like there's a boulder resting on them. You neck and shoulders are always stiff.

You have to be on a low-sodium and a low-sugar diet.

My blood pressure was always on the high side of 220 or more. My doctor always did warn me about stroke but I thought he was just trying to scare me into taking medication.

I was wrongly advised by many so-called supplements experts to try this, take that and even to be a vegetarian. I tried taking some of them for a while. For most cases, it wasn't doing me any good! As for becoming a vegetarian, it wasn't helping too. Maybe due to my prolonged diabetes, nothing was working.

Vegetarian diets were not suitable for me as most of them were high in potassium which are bad for my kidneys and heart.

Once during one of my regular checkups at a nearby Polyclinic, the doctor called for an ambulance to send me to the nearest hospital. I was whisked away from the Polyclinic to the nearest hospital. I was confused, I didn't know what was going on. I was admitted to Alexandra hospital. The doctors there told me my heart almost stopped because the potassium level in my body was extremely high!!!

No two ways about it but never let anyone who does not have the necessary medical training, background or knowledge tell you what you should or shouldn't take!

Weight Loss with the Keto Diet

I decided I could no longer live in this body. My doctor all along has been telling me my main problem was my weight. If I can lose weight, my health will improve.

I decided to take action. I went on a Keto diet. No sugar…no carbohydrates.

Time to say goodbye to soft drinks, rice, noodles, and bread. I even avoided fruits.

I only drank water and ate protein.

I started losing 20kg from 85kg to 65kg. I felt like a brand new person.

I felt good buying clothes that fitted me. The new body felt great for a while.

But the Keto diet did not last. .

When I was hospitalized, the nutritionist asked me about my daily food intake. I told them about the Keto diet. They advised me against it. They said it will do me more harm than good because of my current condition.

Belly Dancing

I love belly dancing. It gave me a level of confidence where I felt good and loved myself more every time I danced. It made me forget my problems.

I was such a natural at belly dancing. By the 4th lesson in the beginner's class, my teacher signed me up for the Master's workshop.

I was shocked to learn all those who attended the Master's workshop were professional dancers and trainers.

Eventually, I became a professional belly dancer. I was offered to teach.

I used belly dancing as a way to help plus size women to love their body and build up their confidence

I loved what I was doing. But the love was short-lived. Within the fraternity, the environment was toxic. There was jealousy, gossips, and bitchiness all around.

I had my glory days as a belly dancer. I used to make lots of money through classes and performance. I became the emcee for belly dance concerts. I was humorous. I was a natural on stage. The crowds loved me. I would perform in some business events. I got contracts and new projects from clients because they were impressed by my belly dancing.

I used to tell my niece "if you want to go far in life, do belly dancing". But for me I think it brought me nothing but destruction.

The diabetes combined with all the years of dancing, took a toll on my feet. My feet are now constantly in pain. After my stroke, I could not walk. I was offered the option to undergo a very painful operation, but the success of the operation is not guaranteed. After the operation if there was an infection…my leg could be amputated.

No thanks, but I am happy with my wheelchair.

Speech Therapy

After the stroke, I suffered loss of speech for two weeks.

For almost half a year, I could not speak without stammering.

Gone are the days when I could speak confidently. I lost my confidence to speak in public. I was invited to speak at a few events but I didn't like what I was hearing. I was not my usual self. I would stutter and stammer. The words and sentences were there in my head but it just seemed impossible to say it out. I would just freeze after a few sentences. It was like my teeth were glued together.

It is a terrible blow to me because I used to make a livelihood as an emcee.

My confidence was so low that I stopped talking to people. I was not comfortable to attend any gatherings because I felt that nobody would understand what I was saying. I had to repeat myself often. I felt so frustrated.

I went for speech therapy. Slowly I recovered. I prayed about it.

The other form of therapy are my two little nieces, who are always jumping around and playing all over me. Sometimes or in fact most of the times, I am forced into role playing with them and all these activities with them has actually helped project my voice. As a result, my speech has improved tremendously. Thanks to my very own two little speech therapists.

Water Retention

Water retention is one of the worst things to go through with.

Kidney disease...Kidney damage...Cirrhosis...Weakness or damage to veins in your legs...these and many more are the known causes for water retention.

Your feet will swell right up to your calves...in fact your whole-body swells. Feels like you've gained weight overnight!

Two minutes of walking and I'll be panting! Feels like I'm dragging a ball and chain!

I'll need to constantly urinate...and every time I stood up to walk, the pain is unbearable...feels like thousands of knives slicing through my legs!

In the middle of the night, my sleep is disrupted because I have to sit up every now and then because of breathlessness!

Doctors recommend that one way of getting rid of the excessive water is by exercising, and so did Mr David Ng who recommended that I take daily walks especially when the weather is hot.

During the night, my throat is always dry but I can't drink anything to quench my thirst as my daily water intake is limited to only 800ml!

To be rid of the water retention, I don't have a choice but to control my water and salt intake too.

For me it's like 'it never rains but it pours' but I'm not giving up anytime soon.

All I can do is hope and pray.

My Love Story

We met when I was running my own cafeteria. He would visit me often at the cafeteria and often after closing for the day, we would go catch a movie or have supper.

As the days went on by, I told him that I was having some health issues and sooner or later I would be a burden to him. I told him that I might go blind. I told him to leave me and look for someone else.

I felt It was very unfair of me to drag him into whatever was coming my way, unfair of me to burden him.

His reply was "why are you so negative, can you be more positive?"

He said he wasn't going anywhere, won't leave me and would stand by me no matter what.

When I had the stroke, he was the first one to rush to the hospital early in the morning. He was there beside me daily from morning till night. He visited me every single day. He stayed by my bed until I fell asleep. He would massage my shoulders, arms and feet every day. He would pray for me. Even asking his family and friends to pray for me.

I told him repeatedly to leave me for a better girlfriend but this macho man with tattoos told me never to talk this way again. He said he would stay with me... period!

God had sent an angel to me. My boyfriend's tender loving care made me love myself again. I do not feel like a handicap anymore. His love healed me. I feel like a Queen now.

What Did I Learn?

What life lessons did I learn during these 3 years of suffering?

Lesson 1: Never self-medicate if you do not know what you are doing. Consult a doctor always!

Lesson 2: Do not listen to salespeople who are not medically qualified. They do not know your medical condition and the effects of the product on your body.

Lesson 3: Understand your food. Food is medicine. Food is also a poison.

Lesson 4: Doctors are fallible too. They are human after all. Always seek a second opinion.

Lesson 5: There is God who is the creator of all things. Reach out to God with your prayers and faith. Nothing is impossible. Believe in Him. Believe in miracles.

Lesson 6: The people who love you will stand by you, support you and strengthen you. Treasure your family, your loved ones and your friends.

Lesson 7: Do good. Karma repays your kindness manifold.

Lesson 8: Money is important. But it is not everything. There are many things that money can buy. But it cannot buy you happiness, peace of mind, health, or love.

Lesson 9: Don't worry too much. Worrying is a waste of time. To worry is like sitting on a rocking chair…It keeps you busy in motion but you are not moving anywhere.

Lesson 10: Trials and tribulation bring us closer to God. It is a gift.

Lesson 11: Be patient. Your body can heal itself. Give it time.

The Road Ahead

Every day, I am still in pain physically and emotionally.

I want to live without pain.

I want to walk, I want to run.

I want to sleep in my bed, not in a hospital bed.

I want to be well and live like a normal human being again.

I want to get married and have a house of my own.

I want to bring my mother out of the nursing home and give her the first-class care that she deserves. I want to take care of her for the rest of her life.

I want to keep fit by eating healthy food and exercising regularly. Health is wealth!

I want to share my message with the world, a message of hope that sickness can be treated. I want to alert the public not to make the same mistakes I made.

** The End **

www.ingramcontent.com/pod-product-compliance
Lightning Source LLC
Chambersburg PA
CBHW072018280526
45788CB00007B/2603